How To Deal With Dementia Patient

The Ultimate Guide On How To Handle Dementia Patients

Stephanie Mike

Table of Contents

Chapter 1

Understanding Dementia

Dementia sufferers, as well as their families and loved ones, can face tough conditions. As dementia progresses, the patient may begin to function in ways that are unknown to them, causing their behavior to shift radically.

This can be challenging for family caregivers to handle since behavioral changes typically occur unexpectedly, and it takes time to identify what is generating them. Even though families frequently find it difficult to accept a loved one's dementia diagnosis, managing challenging behavior might become less difficult over time.

Contrary to common opinion, dementia is not a single medical disorder, but rather a handy umbrella word for a variety of distinct diseases. They all have one thing in common: they are associated with cognitive decline. Depending on the patient's state, certain areas of the brain begin to lose their usual function. This is commonly caused by brain cell death or protein bodies impeding neuronal connections.

Symptoms of dementia may include:

- *Confusion and disorientation.*

- *Decreased coordination with motor functions.*

- *Depression, Anxiety, Paranoia, and Agitation*

- *Difficulty managing complex activities, critical thinking abilities, planning, and organization.*

- *Difficulty with linguistic expressiveness.*

- *Hallucinations*

- *Inappropriate behaviour*

* *Memory loss.*

* *Personality changes.*

* *Challenges with visual or spatial abilities*

* *Struggling with problem-solving or reasoning*

Alzheimer's is the most frequent type of dementia. This disorder is caused by the creation of disruptive protein complexes that block linked brain cells, resulting in their death. The signs of Alzheimer's disease may include:

* *Apathy and Depression*

* *Personality changes such as disinterest, distrust, and hostility*

* *Confusion*

* *Difficulty concentrating*

* *Difficulty speaking, swallowing, or walking*

* *Impaired judgment or decision-making ability*

* *Mood shifts.*

* *Having problems remembering specifics about people, places, or occasions.*

Many of these symptoms are shared with other types of dementia, but they warrant special attention because Alzheimer's accounts for around 70% of all dementia cases.

Dementia symptoms are very challenging for patients and family members to deal with because they are unlike most other illnesses. Because of the cognitive and psychological character of dementia, patients are prone to alterations in their thinking and behavior. This can be a very unsettling sensation, leading to disruptive or even hostile behavior.

As you begin to notice dementia behaviors, keep in mind that these are not your loved one's intentional choice, but rather an unpleasant side consequence of their disease. Managing dementia behaviors can be tough for family members because their loved one is often not acting like the person they have always known, which can cause distress.

Understanding what dementia behavior is and then establishing ways to control it effectively can be extremely beneficial.

Chapter 2

Creating a Safe and Comfortable Environment

When a loved one is diagnosed with dementia, families are frequently faced with the difficult dilemma of whether to provide home care or residential care. Many persons with dementia can live peacefully and safely at home for a while after making certain changes to their living environment and daily routines. However, if the illness worsens, symptoms such as memory loss, confusion, and unstable mobility can make independent living more dangerous.

Caring for someone with dementia at home requires adapting to their changing demands. This allows them to maintain as much freedom as possible while simultaneously protecting them from falls, accidents, and wandering hazards.

Noise levels

Background noise can impair a person with dementia's ability to concentrate or process information. Turn off the television or radio if they are not in use, especially if you are attempting to have a discussion. Soft furniture, like rugs and cushions, can assist in absorbing and reducing unwanted noises, such as the sound of someone walking across a room or closing a door.

Disengaging the doorbell may also be a smart precaution if sudden loud noises are particularly unsettling; replacing it with a video doorbell may be a better alternative.

Furniture and fittings

Dementia can make people feel disoriented, even in familiar surroundings, and specific shapes and patterns can exacerbate this confusion. They may also struggle to recognize themselves in the mirror, which can be extremely painful. As a result, some people remove or conceal mirrors in their homes until needed.

If you need to make any of the adjustments described below, try not to change the arrangement of a room too much at once, as this may have the opposite impact.

Striped or bold patterned furnishings should be removed or covered to avoid confusion.

Use bold, contrasting colors to easily identify chairs and tables from walls and floors.

Add a chair with arms that are simpler to rise from.

Entertainment

Television can be a great source of companionship and enjoyment, but you should regulate its use and encourage a person with dementia to watch something lighter or shorter. This could include gaming shows, nostalgic or familiar comedy, nature documentaries, or shows centered on hobbies or interests.

News and current affairs broadcasts may induce distress if the viewer is unable to digest the information presented. Even if they don't fully comprehend what's being said, persons with dementia may detect the tone of a program.

Simplify and declutter

A cluttered, chaotic environment is too exciting for someone with dementia, it can lead to confusion, anxiety, and agitation. Go through each area and remove any unneeded furniture and accessories. Remove patterned wallpaper and flooring if possible, as busy designs are frequently viewed as barriers by dementia patients. Stick to solid, neutral colors that are soothing and unobtrusive.

Improve lighting

Install appropriate illumination throughout the home, with light switches in convenient locations. Consider installing motion-sensor night lights in corridors and restrooms to avoid falls during nighttime wanderings. Check for any shadows or glare that may induce misperceptions. During the day, open your blinds and drapes to allow natural light in, which helps regulate your circadian cycles.

Support independent toileting
Incontinence is common with dementia, but accidents can be reduced with some easy adjustments. Place colorful posters or images on restroom doors to aid identification. Install grab bars, nonslip matting, and an elevated toilet seat to improve stability. Install a motion sensor or magnetic light that goes on automatically when the bathroom door opens at nighttime.

Keep the essentials within reach
To reduce frustration, keep regularly used items such as glasses, slippers, and medication in easily accessible locations. You can also use words or graphics to label drawers and cabinets. Replace knobs with easy-to-use levers on doors and taps. Simple repairs should be completed immediately to avoid potential mishaps.

Laundries
Laundries should be as straightforward and familiar as feasible. If you need to make modifications, consider keeping the benches tidy or labeling the cupboards to make things easier to find.

If the individual with dementia can no longer use the washing machines safely, consider removing cleaning chemicals and poisons, storing the iron in a locked cupboard, and turning the washing machine and dryer off at the wall. Make sure electrical connections are not in contact with water or heating sources.

Supporting memory
Memory loss is a typical sign of dementia and can be particularly upsetting. There are numerous techniques to help someone remember things and find their way around. Consider what types of items the person with dementia typically forgets. This will assist you in determining which memory aids to utilize.

For example, if they have difficulties remembering to do their chores, post a whiteboard in a prominent spot, such as beside the refrigerator, and write daily task lists on it. If they frequently misplace their keys, keep them in the same location every day and post reminders throughout the house.

Placing photos and familiar things about the home helps people with dementia keep linked to their history. Using easy-to-read clocks or huge calendars around the house helps children stay in the present.

Outdoor places

It is important that outdoor spaces be peaceful, safe, and quiet for individuals with dementia to stroll through. For example, you could install a raised garden bed that kids could plant and care for. Set timers on hoses to water the garden without the user having to remember to turn off the tap when they're done.

Many people with dementia find comfort and companionship in their pets, but it's important to make sure the animal is well-cared for and unable to escape.

You might need to adjust and lock the gates. You may even need to put up fences but exercise caution because a new fence might make a person with dementia feel trapped.

Take into consideration clearing out anything in the way of walks, hiding trash or compost bins, getting rid of any poisonous or spiky plants, and putting away any dangerous chemicals in the garage or garden shed, if you have any.

Kitchens

Kitchens should be safe and allow people to use them independently for as long as possible. Try to keep everything familiar and avoid rearranging too many items. If possible, replace an appliance with the same make and model. Appliances with built-in safety measures, such as a kettle with an automatic shut-off switch, are an excellent choice. Keep electrical wires away from water and heating sources.

It may be helpful to label cupboards to make things easier to find or keep frequently used goods on the bench.

If the person is no longer able to use the kitchen safely, you may need to install a master shut-off switch for the stove and remove any sharp blades, medicines, or poisonous chemicals. Reduce the temperature of the hot water tap, and have a list of contact names and numbers in large type near the phone.

Dementia-friendly home products
There are home goods available that are specifically developed for people with dementia. For example:

Clocks with big LCD displays indicate the day, date, and time.

Telephones with large buttons

Reminder devices that provide an audio cue to assist individuals in remembering to take their medications or secure the front door

These products are often referred to as assistive technology. Apps for cell phones and tablets are also useful. A number of websites, such as Living Made Easy and the Alzheimer's Society online store, offer daily living help. You may discover that the person you care for enjoys classic fixtures and fittings, such as taps, toilet flushes, and bath plugs.

Make sure all tables are stable and have round, smooth edges. They should be at an appropriate height to allow for the visibility of food and drink, as well as the ability to put a wheelchair below.

Use technology to increase safety
Specialist technology is available to let people live independently while still monitoring their safety. Motion sensors, door alarms, and bed alarms can notify caretakers if a dementia patient moves around at unexpected times. Location devices enable tracking if the person wanders away from home. Automated drug dispensers send

warnings and reminders. Consider installing one or more of these
devices to provide peace of mind.

Chapter 3

Effective Communication Strategies

For individuals suffering from dementia, their loved ones, and caretakers, losing the ability to communicate can be among the most upsetting and challenging problems. As the disease develops, the individual with dementia increasingly loses their ability to communicate. They are finding it increasingly challenging to express themselves accurately and understand what others are saying.

It is critical to ensure that communication difficulties are not due to compromised vision or hearing. Some people may benefit from wearing glasses or using a hearing aid. Make sure your hearing aids work properly and that your glasses are cleaned on a regular basis.

Every individual with dementia is unique, and the problems in articulating thoughts and feelings vary. Dementia has several origins, each of which affects the brain in a distinct way.

Some changes you could see in the person with dementia are:

- *Difficulty locating a word; a related word may be offered instead of one they cannot recall.*
- *Nonsensical speech*
- *An inability to grasp what you are saying or the ability to merely grasp a portion of what you are saying.*
- *Writing and reading skills have worsened*
- *Loss of typical conversational customs, an increased inclination to interrupt, disregard a speaker, or fail to answer when spoken to*
- *Difficulty expressing emotions effectively.*

Communicating with someone with dementia

Caregivers must consider how they show themselves to the person with dementia. The three components that comprise the messages we communicate are:

- *Body language accounts for 55% of communication.*
- *The tone and pitch of our voices, which accounts for 38% of communication*
- *The words we use account for 7% of conversation.*

These figures emphasize the significance of how relatives and caregivers portray themselves to someone with dementia. Raised eyebrows and sighs are examples of negative body language that is easily picked up on. There are several tactics or approaches you can use to communicate effectively with someone with dementia, make yourself known, and demonstrate your concern for them.

Caring attitude

Because people still feel things even when they don't understand what is being said, it's important to maintain their dignity and sense of worth. Be flexible and give yourself plenty of time to hear back. Touch can be used to keep someone's attention and to express warmth and compassion when it's suitable.

Ways of speaking

When communicating with a person with dementia, attempt to:

- *Keep sentences brief and straightforward, and focus on one idea at a time.*
- *Always provide enough time for what you've stated to be understood.*
- *Remain calm and speak in a pleasant, matter-of-fact manner.*

Body Language

You may need to utilize hand gestures and facial expressions to communicate. Pointing and demonstrating can help. Touching and holding the person's hand might assist keep their attention and demonstrate that you care. A pleasant grin and shared laughter can often express more than words.

The right environment.
When speaking with someone who has dementia, attempt to:

- ❖ *Avoid competing noises, such as TV and radio.*

- ❖ *Stay stationary while talking; this makes it easier for the person with dementia to understand what you're saying*

- ❖ *Maintaining consistent habits might help to reduce confusion and improve communication.*

Maintain a consistent approach; utilizing the same communication style will make it far less confusing for the person with dementia. Repeating the message in the same way is critical for all family members and caregivers.

What Not to Do
- ❖ *Instead of telling the person what they cannot do, say what they can do.*

- ❖ *A condescending tone of speech can be picked up, even if the words are not understood.*

- ❖ *Ask a lot of direct questions that require a solid memory.*

- ❖ *Talk about the persons in front of them as if they were not present.*

- ❖ *Avoid arguing with the person since it will worsen the situation. Instead, order them about.*

Therapies and Communication Strategies

There are a number of different communication styles that have been developed in an effort to provide someone the support and trust they need to be well. Many family members and caregivers will use some of these approaches spontaneously without knowing their formal names.

Validation Therapy with Dementia

Validation therapy explains that instead of attempting to return the person with dementia to our reality, it is more beneficial to enter their reality. This allows you to generate empathy for the person while also establishing trust and security. This, in turn, lowers anxiety.

For instance, family and caregivers that use validation would not dispute or insist that their loved one understand their actions if the person with dementia thinks she is waiting for her now middle-aged children to get home from school. They declined to correct the dementia sufferer's opinions.

Instead, using the validating technique, caregivers would identify and empathize with the emotions underlying the behavior being displayed. This ensures that the individual with dementia retains their dignity and self-esteem.

Reminiscence and Dementia

Reminiscence is the process of reviewing past occurrences. This is typically a highly positive and satisfying activity. Even if the person with dementia is unable to communicate vocally, they can still enjoy reminiscing and reflecting on the past. It might also serve as a distraction if the individual feels upset.

While reflecting on past events might bring a sense of calm and enjoyment, it can also evoke unpleasant and sad emotions. It is critical to be sensitive to the person's reactions if this occurs. If their distress appears overpowering, it is preferable to employ another sort of diversion to alleviate worry.

"This is Your Life" book and Dementia

Creating a chronological history of the person with dementia might aid with reminiscence and provide information to those who may engage with them. It can also assist carers visiting the home or residential care facility in learning more about the individual and their lives. A This Is Your Life or Memory Book is a visual diary that functions similarly to a family photo album. It may comprise letters, postcards, certificates, and other souvenirs.

A huge photo album with plastic protection sheets on each page can survive extensive use. Each photo must be labeled to prevent putting the person with dementia on the spot with inquiries like 'Who is that?'. It is advisable to limit the content on each page to one topic and no more than two or three items.

Music Therapy and Dementia
Music-related activities are another great technique to communicate with someone with dementia. Even when other abilities have faded, the individual can still enjoy old familiar melodies and tunes. A particular piece of music can evoke memories and emotions. It is critical to be ready to respond to the release of these emotions.

Knowing a person's musical preferences and dislikes is critical for this to be an effective strategy. Music can be utilized for formal therapeutic or recreational purposes. It can also assist in the management of challenging behaviors. Music therapists have received training in the use of music with patients with dementia and can handle some extremely complicated behaviors.

Chapter 4

Daily Care Routines

In the early stages of the disease, daily routines assist persons with dementia navigate their surroundings in a predictable manner and offer a sense of order to their days, which becomes even more crucial as they lose awareness of time. Furthermore, because routines are kept in long-term memory, while dementia typically affects short-term memory first, routines are frequently accessible even in the later stages of the disease.

People with dementia struggle to learn new things because they have short-term memory loss. They may have difficulty remembering instructions or staying concentrated for longer periods of time. Daily routines assist persons with dementia cope with the symptoms of short-term memory loss by immersing them in familiar tasks. Because they know they will soon lose the ability to perform numerous daily duties, continuing to do them for as long as possible becomes critical. It fosters a sense of independence, boosts self-esteem, and may even help kids retain skills for longer.

Another key benefit of a daily routine for dementia sufferers is reduced anxiety. As the disease progresses, dementia patients grow increasingly dissatisfied with their loss of cognitive and physical capacities. Routines can help them approach the day with a stronger sense of calm and security, reducing agitation and disruptive conduct.

Establishing daily routines can also assist caregivers reduce stress, which is equally vital. Days frequently run more smoothly when a more regular environment and routine are established. When a person with dementia is less agitated, there are greater chances for moments of joy and connection.

Tips for Creating Daily Routine

The following are some useful guidelines and strategies for creating a daily routine when caring for someone with dementia.

Customise routines to their preferences.
This is not the time to make substantial changes in their environment. Maintain routines that mirror the majority of the dementia patient's life experiences. Maintain a consistent regimen, such as brushing their teeth before breakfast or eating ice cream after supper.

Maintain your ability to adapt.
Recognize that as the condition worsens, your talents will change. It's critical to remain adaptable and tweak the routine to accommodate these changes while still allowing your loved one to do as much as they can. This may take longer than completing everything alone, but patience is essential and will promote a sense of independence and accomplishment. Also, if they appear bored or irritated, consider changing the activity or taking a break.

Allow them to help.
To help the person with dementia retain cognitive and motor abilities, involve them in daily domestic duties such as cleaning dishes or folding laundry. Even if they don't get the dishes entirely clean or fold the clothes perfectly, let them do it without being corrected. Praise them for their assistance to boost their self-esteem, then proceed to the next portion of the exercise.

Make dull daily tasks part of the routine.
Simple actions like constantly setting their meds next to their beverage at breakfast, bathing in the morning or at night, getting dressed, and so on help reinforce a feeling of order and purpose.

Physical activity.
This can be as basic as going for a stroll at a specific time of day when the weather is pleasant or performing chair yoga together when you are unable to get outside.

Time activity

Even if the person with dementia is oblivious to the time on the clock, establishing routines that provide indications as to the time of day or day of the week can help boost feelings of security. For example, do they usually watch a favorite television show on a specific day or time? Do they appreciate a Sunday afternoon meal? Make such things a part of your routine. You can also utilize clues like raising the curtains in the morning and closing them at night, arranging the table before dinner, lowering the lights, or pulling back the bedcovers when it's time for bed. These nonverbal cues will become increasingly crucial as your loved one's ability to process speech deteriorates.

Therapeutic Activity

Do they appreciate arts & crafts or other visual challenges, like puzzles? Have they always had a garden or kept an excellent lawn? While they may not be able to till the soil or drive a lawn mower, they may be able to plant seeds, water a garden, and pluck weeds. Choose activities that are safe and appropriate for their skills so that they can continue to appreciate the things that have always given them pleasure.

Music in their day.

According to research, music provides numerous benefits for people with dementia, in part because musical appreciation and ability are among the last abilities to be lost. Listening to music can elicit feelings and memories, and music associated with a specific activity can assist a person with dementia in remembering the action. If it is physically feasible, dancing to music can help people with dementia express their feelings. Additionally, being physically close to someone while dancing might provide them with a sense of security. Researchers also discovered that singing activated the left side of the brain while listening to music stimulated the right, and watching the [singing] class activated visual sections of the brain.

Consider their needs when arranging a trip or holiday.
If you wish to take a vacation with a person with dementia, find a
destination that they are familiar with. For example, does your family
always go to the same beach in the summer or the same mountain
chalet in the fall? While familiar surroundings may calm your loved
one and perhaps recall memories, visiting a completely new location
may cause anxiety and restlessness.

It is unavoidable that some disruptions to the routine will occur,
whether it is a medical appointment for a person with dementia, your
own appointment, your becoming ill, or simply needing a few days
off. Recall that the daily schedule is only meant to give structure to
the day; it does not need to be strict when taking care of someone
who has dementia.

Chapter 5

Managing Behavior Changes

Using comforting language to meet needs, changing locations, and engaging in calming activities are all effective ways of dealing with undesired behaviors.

Agitation is the leading reason Americans place loved ones with dementia in care facilities. More than 5 million Americans have dementia, and 80% of them may experience behavioral symptoms such as aggressiveness, hallucinations, or delusions at some point.

As the older population expands, healthcare practitioners may encounter more distressed caregivers of dementia patients seeking assistance in managing problematic behaviors. Though the majority of agitation is most likely caused by deteriorating conditions, healthcare personnel can affect behaviors.

Why Behaviors Occur
Some experts argue that all behaviors are kinds of communication. When the disease has deprived a patient of language and reasoning, perplexing or "bad" behavior may be an attempt to communicate an unmet need. Resistance-type behaviors may be a reaction to a loss of control, bewilderment about what is going on, or even a sense of urgency in any given situation. A patient may be depressed, in pain, or experiencing stress. It is believed that when the neurological system degenerates, patients' ability to cope with stress declines.

Detective Work
To sort through patients' behavioral cues, caregivers must be patient and persistent. They should start by ruling out obvious physical causes such as pain, injury, constipation, infection, damp briefs, tight or uncomfortable clothing, or a patient feeling too hot or cold.

A patient may provide information about an underlying condition. In one case, a patient complained bitterly that his foot hurt. An emergency department examination indicated a serious bladder infection. Following therapy, the patient reported that his foot was no longer pained. He had provided the most important indication, that he was in pain, and it was up to caregivers and health care specialists to determine the source.

Caregivers should analyze the previous day's events to determine whether a patient is weary from a lack of sleep or whether there have been any changes to a patient's routine or environment, such as the presence of basic holiday decorations. People suffering from dementia are afraid of change.

Triggers
Experts in dementia have identified six factors that frequently cause agitation: weariness, change, a sense of loss, amount of stimulation, excessive demands, and physical stresses such as pain, infections, or constipation.

Agitation and Aggression
Agitation, restlessness, and anxiety are all frequent in dementia patients, but violence is especially concerning. These behaviors can start abruptly or develop out of a patient's frustration. The key to managing them is to investigate the origins of the behaviors in order to understand the sentiments that motivate the actions.

After evaluating for physical discomforts, investigate what occurred immediately preceding the unfavorable behavior. What sparked it? Taking the time to sort this out could help prevent future instances. Address the patient using a calm, soothing tone and reassurance, such as "You appear upset. I'm sorry you're angry, but I am right here. Let's get some cookies.

Try a different setting, something unexpected or diverting, such as dancing, singing a song, going for a stroll, or just moving to another room. Engage the patient in a creative endeavor or ask for help with a chore. Take a ride in the automobile. Play popular hymns,

Christmas carols, and old-time music. Keep in mind that reasoning does not work.

Wandering

Approximately two-thirds of individuals with dementia will wander at some point. Be prepared. A patient might stray when looking for someone, "going to work," relieving frustration, or looking for a restaurant. Identifying the cause of wandering may provide insight into how to manage it. The following measures can help eliminate or lessen a dementia patient's inclination to wander:

A large black mat in front of or just situated outside a door may look to the patient as a gaping hole that cannot be passed.

Inform your neighbors about their wandering tendencies and provide them with contact information.

Make the patient wear an ID bracelet provided by MedicAlert or the Alzheimer's Association. Consider using a GPS wristband built specifically for this purpose.

Have a recent photograph to show if a patient wanders.

Involve the person in daily duties such as folding towels, drying dishes, or putting out the trash. This will help you sleep better, feel more in control, and lessen your worry.

Encourage physical activity by going for a stroll, dancing, or exercising together.

Install deadbolts or key-operated locks to improve house safety. Never lock a dementia patient at home alone. Put child-safe covers on outside doorknobs.

Cover the entrance with a curtain or a full-length image of a bookcase. Other signs that dissuade a patient from approaching a door include STOP! and DO NOT ENTER.

Suspicion or Paranoia

Many patients with dementia go through this period. They may assume that someone is attempting to steal their money or possessions. This feels extremely real to dementia patients; explaining and reasoning will not help. This is not a reflection of the patient's thoughts; rather, it is a medical symptom.

Allow the person to speak without correcting them. Be reassuring, telling him or her who you are and that you are there to help, using statements like "Let me help you hunt for the money," and subsequently drawing attention to a picture album in the space. If money is a persistent problem, save coins and tiny notes in your purse or wallet to "discover" in the future. If a person suspects someone is breaking into the house, soothe him or her with words such as, "That must be frightening. I am right here. "I'll make sure nothing bad happens to you." Refocus your attention.

Sundown Syndrome

Sundowning is a word that describes heightened disorientation and perplex in the late afternoon and early evening. Sundown syndrome is experienced by up to 20% of adults with dementia. This behavior is usually most severe in the middle stages of Alzheimer's disease and decreases as the disease progresses.

Symptoms of sundown syndrome include mood swings, irritation, screaming, lashing out at caretakers, pacing, tremors, and suspicion. As shadows appear, they may have trouble sleeping, wander more, and "wish to go home." They may be aware of their own perplexity, which might cause more aggravation.

Alzheimer's disease appears to alter the brain's regulation of sleep and wakefulness patterns. Other possible causes include mental and physical exhaustion; low lighting and increased shadows; discomfort caused by pain, urinary tract infection, fecal impaction, and so on; medications; hunger; a sleep environment that is too noisy; an absence of planned evening activities; sleeping excessively throughout the day; or people coming and going.

Use encouraging phrases, such as "You'll be fine. You're in a safe place; not arguing with or correcting him or her; looking for unmet needs such as cold, hungry, wet, or in pain; moving him or her to a quieter, more serene area, like the bedroom; keeping them occupied with a favorite activity around the time when dusk usually falls, such as enlisting help to make dinner, completing an art project or having a bath, whichever the person enjoys doing; and remembering past bedtime rituals.

Consider alternative techniques such as aromatherapy, pets, calming white noise, like ocean waves or crickets, calming cuisine, hand massages, reading aloud from beloved poetry, singing, or brushing their hair; several of these methods can be used simultaneously.

Sleep Problems
Many persons with dementia struggle with their circadian rhythms, which control their sleep and wake states. Some tips to help normalize keeping regular sleep and daily routines, restricting daytime naps to 15 to 20 minutes, and increasing daytime exercise, such as walking or dancing, are examples of good sleep habits. Steer clear of caffeine or limit its consumption to the morning; provide a small snack before bed to avoid hunger being a source of irritation; and allow maximum autonomy in making decisions, including choosing one's favorite place to sleep.

If none of these measures work, seek medical counsel. Medical issues may be causing the confusion and agitation at night. A physician can also assess a patient's drugs, removing any that cause problems or are unnecessary.

Bathing
Bathing can cause agitation in dementia sufferers. It may feel weird for a person with dementia to have assistance with an activity that he or she has always done alone. Making plans in advance might be quite advantageous.

First, treat the pain. If the patient has pain when moving, medication at least 30 to 60 minutes before the bath. Prepare all of your supplies in advance. Explain your plans and assuage any anxieties. Maintain modesty while ensuring that the room and water temperature are pleasant.

Make bathing a joyful spa experience. A patient may eventually come to like bathing. Play your favorite music, provide food or beverage, use aromatherapy, or apply your favorite perfume or aftershave. Give a shoulder rub. Find appealing techniques to engage all of the patient's senses.

Allow the patient to accomplish as much as possible for themselves. Giving people alternatives restores their sense of control at a time when they have lost so much. Give choices, like "Do you want me to help you wash your face or would you rather I do it yourself?

Sustaining regular routines, especially a regular bath routine, is essential for sustaining serenity. Agitation can result from surprise or rushing a person suffering from dementia.

Sexual Behaviors
One of the core human needs is the desire for closeness. People with dementia continue to require loving, safe connections and caring touches. Sexuality is one way to communicate that urge.

While some dementia sufferers lose interest in sexual activity, others may still desire it. Patients with dementia may exhibit inappropriate sexual behaviors, such as undressing, fondling, or making inappropriate sexual advances when their inhibitions wear off.

Remember that inappropriate behavior is a result of the sickness, not a reflection of the individual. A person with dementia may not understand how to properly channel sexual urges or when to express a desire for physical love.

Don't be scared or shame the individual. Walk him or her to a secluded space. This is a wonderful opportunity to use distraction strategies, such as giving a special treat, introducing a favorite object, or scheduling time with a pet.

During the day, make physical touch by holding hands, brushing someone's hair, or offering a back rub.

Communication

Simple things can significantly improve communication with a dementia sufferer. For instance, are his or her glasses clean, hearing aids in position, and the batteries in the hearing aids new? Find a location distant from distractions like television or radio. If necessary, close the curtains or the door.

Concentrate on your communication style. Sit down, if feasible, at the person's eye level; standing over someone might be intimidating. If you think the patient may have forgotten who you are, introduce yourself. Speak in a friendly tone and smile. Speak gently, calmly, and clearly, not any louder. Do not fight or reason with the person; rationality does not help.

Speak in brief sentences, pausing after each to allow the listener to comprehend what you've said. Provide one straightforward lesson at a time. When a dementia patient is urged to "put on your shoes and socks, clean your teeth, comb your hair, and come to the kitchen to have your breakfast," none of those things may happen. Use hand gestures wherever possible, such as patting the chair where you wish the guest to sit. Wait patiently for a response before repeating yourself.

Delirium

In contrast to dementia, which is a long-term condition, delirium is distinguished by an abrupt shift in mental capacity. Delirium is curable and should be addressed immediately. If non-drug therapy fails, antipsychotics may be useful. Delirium is defined by a quick change in mental abilities, inability to focus or sustain attention, altered perception of surroundings, disorganized behavior, unpredictable or fluctuating status, and a sudden start within hours or days.

A new or changing environment, such as hospitalization, electrolyte imbalance, fecal impaction, urine retention, drug interactions or side effects, pain, stress, injury, or a significant medical problem, such as a stroke, organ failure, or blood clot, can all cause delirium.

Delirium, like agitation, may frequently be avoided or reversed by providing a peaceful, familiar environment and routines, activities during the day and quiet surroundings at night, working glasses and hearing aids, and relaxing techniques such as music, massage, or reading to the patient.

Rummage Bags
People suffering from dementia frequently experience a sense of loss, including possessions, memory, and the capacity to speak. The feeling of having lost something might generate anxiety or uneasiness. A rummage bag is a tool for occupying, distracting, and satisfying a dementia patient with an activity that is relevant to how they are feeling. It can also alleviate boredom.

Use a large purse, a men's toiletry bag, or any other bag containing a variety of familiar objects that may be enjoyable to touch, move, or study. It can be readily filled with basic household items. Avoid things small enough to ingest, sharp objects, and anything that can be disassembled. Be inventive. A bag could include goods such as the keys, contact book, wallet, indestructible mirror, coin purse, tiny stuffed animal, non-sharp kitchen utensils, sample credit cards, pictures, TV remote without battery power, comb, casino chips, old mobile phone, sealed flashlight, or a bottle opening device.

Distraction Kit
Create a bag or box of fascinating, unusual, and enjoyable activities to use when you need to divert someone's attention. Eventually, the box may have such positive memories that the patient swiftly shifts his or her focus to it. It could contain aromatherapy or perfume; a sound machine that plays chirping, rain, waves, and other noises; picture books, a music box, hand or foot massage cream, and a cozy flannel blanket in the dryer and wrap around feet; or special goodies.

Chapter 6

Activities & Engagement

One technique to keep dementia patients motivated is to explore their previous interests or talents. Explore the following activities to rekindle a loved one's former hobbies and strengths.

Experiment with sound
Music has a significant impact on people with dementia, sparking memories and fostering creativity. Introducing modest musical instruments or songs might provide enjoyable experiences for individuals with dementia.

Encourage visual expression
Painting and drawing are safe and creative ways to express one's feelings. Encourage the use of bold, vivid colors on large surfaces. Rolls of butcher paper allow seniors with dementia to create without the stress of confined surroundings. These types of visual exercises for dementia sufferers are not only enjoyable but also therapeutic, as they encourage emotional expression.

Investigate sensory craft activities
Activities with diverse textures, such as playing with clay, provide tactile stimulation to dementia patients. Using these resources to create crafts or just to experiment with different sizes and shapes can be enjoyable and helpful.

Create collages
Cut out photos from magazines or print old advertisements and articles. Choose topics that correspond to your loved one's passions, such as cooking, cars, or fashion. Reproducing ancient family photos digitally is an additional option. Allow your family member with dementia to arrange and rearrange the materials to make photos or scrapbook pages.

Chapter 7

Emotional Support for Caregivers

Caregiver stress is a natural element of dementia caregiving. There are things you may take to alleviate it, but first, you must acknowledge it. These include denial that the individual has dementia, rage toward the person with dementia and others, emotional sensitivity, social retreat, and depression. Symptoms include a lack of sleep, difficulty concentrating, tiredness, anxiety, and an increase in health issues. Here are a few things caregivers may do to make their lives easier:

❖ *People who are stressed should see their doctor on a regular basis.*

❖ *Seek support from family and friends.*

❖ *Take advantage of community services that offer respite and relief from caregiving, practical aid with meals or cleaning, and support for the person with dementia.*

❖ *Also, plan ahead for both the current and long-term.*

Supporting a person with dementia takes time and effort. It can be a great experience, but it can also be difficult and frustrating. Knowing and recognizing stress symptoms in yourself or someone you care about is the first step toward taking action.

Ways to Reduce Caregiver Stress

Remain realistic about dementia
It is crucial, while tough, to be honest about dementia and how it will affect the individual over time. Being realistic will make it easy to change your expectations.

Be realistic about yourself

You need to be realistic about your abilities. What do you value the most? A walk with the person you're caring for, time alone, or a clean house? There is no "correct" response; only you know what is important to you and how much you can contribute.

Accept your feelings

You will experience a wide range of emotions when caring for someone with dementia. In a single day, you may feel satisfied, angry, guilty, joyful, sad, ashamed, terrified, or helpless. These emotions may be perplexing. But they're typical. Recognize that you're doing your best.

Share your thoughts and feelings with others

Sharing information on dementia with family and friends will help them understand what is going on and prepare them to provide the assistance and support they require. It is equally necessary to express your emotions. Locate a person you can talk about your feelings with without feeling awkward. This could be a close friend or family member, someone you met at a support group, a member of your religious community, or a healthcare professional.

Be positive

Your attitude might influence the way you feel, and try to look at the bright side of things. It can be helpful to focus on what the person can do rather than what talents have been lost. Try to make each day count. There can still be instances that are memorable and fulfilling.

Look for humor

While dementia is a terrible condition, there may be some positive aspects to specific scenarios. Maintaining a sense of humor can be an effective coping tactic.

Take care of yourself

Your health is crucial. Don't disregard it. Consume healthfully and do regular exercise. Find ways to unwind and get the rest you need. Make regular doctor's appointments for check-ups. You should also take regular breaks from caregiving. Do not wait until you are really exhausted to plan this. Take the time to maintain your interests and hobbies. Keep in touch with your friends and family to avoid feeling lonely and isolated. These items will give you the strength to keep offering care.

Get help

Sharing your thoughts and feelings with others will provide you with the necessary support. This could occur alone, with a professional, or as part of a dementia support group. Choose the type of support that makes you the most comfortable. Practical help: It can be difficult to ask for and accept support. However, asking for assistance does not indicate inadequate caregiving. You cannot care for a dementia patient alone. Seek aid from family and friends. Most individuals will be willing to help you. Programs in your neighborhood may provide assistance with household chores or caring duties. Your local Alzheimer's Society can assist you get access to these.

Plan for the future

Planning for the future can assist in reducing stress. If possible, discuss finances with the person with dementia and plan properly. Choices about future health and personal care should be discussed and documented. Legal and estate planning should also be addressed. Consider creating an alternate caregiving plan in case you are unable to give care in the future.

Conclusion

Being a caretaker for a loved one is both extremely rewarding and tough. It can be really challenging to care for a loved one who has dementia.

Dementia refers to a widespread deterioration in cognitive function. There are numerous forms, including Alzheimer's disease, Lewy body dementia, and frontotemporal dementia, to mention a few. Each type of dementia has its own distinguishing qualities. What all varieties have in common is growing cognitive deterioration, which makes daily functioning increasingly challenging.

As a result, persons with dementia require a caregiver to help them with daily duties and personal care, as well as make decisions about their health, finances, and other issues.

Dementia can cause memory problems, decreased decision-making, and behavioral changes, so caring for someone with dementia can be both psychologically and physically demanding. However, you must always keep in mind that you are not alone. There is aid and resources available for you and your loved one. Here are five tips for caring for someone with dementia.

New modes of interaction and communication
It's easy to see a parent or loved one with dementia as they always have been. However, it is crucial to recognize that he or she is now a distinct person. They may appear to be the same, but their behaviors will alter, and you will not be able to return them to normal via pure effort alone. Instead, take measures to change your perception, interaction, and communication with your loved one.

Being willing to accept them as they are today will help you better interact with them in your daily activities. It can also help you understand how to properly respond to the difficult situations that will undoubtedly emerge, such as constantly asking the same question, forgetting something crucial, or acting inappropriately.

It is vital that you provide your loved one plenty of grace; if you find yourself becoming irritated or short-tempered, remind yourself that they are not doing these things purposefully. Their acts and attitudes are the outcome of circumstances beyond their control.

Take measures to prevent agitation, tension, and confrontation
Dementia weakens the brain's ability to handle stress and confusion. As much as feasible, support your loved one succeed by limiting situations that cause conflict or unneeded change.

Tough talks and circumstances will emerge; however, avoid unnecessary conflict and try not to magnify minor everyday issues. Getting into an argument with your loved one isn't fair to them, so instead focus your efforts on dissolving these situations.

The brain likes patterns; the more it understands its environment and routine, the better it can perform. When caring for someone with dementia, it is critical to work with rather than against their strength. You can accomplish this by sticking to a typical routine as much as possible. Avoid introducing your loved one to unfamiliar situations too frequently or recklessly. Keep them as close to their normal habitat as possible.

Recognize unsafe conditions and take measures
Impaired memory or decision-making might make some circumstances dangerous for your loved one. You, as the caregiver, must notice safety concerns and act quickly to address them.

The particular precautions required to keep your loved one safe will most likely be highly individualized and dependent on the unique characteristics of their dementia. However, there are several frequent issues to be aware of, such as driving a car and using some kitchen equipment. Knowing the potential hazards in your loved one's house and taking precautions to make them safer.

Cooking on the stove can be risky for folks who are forgetful, but using the microwave may be safer. Allowing folks who get lost easily or have difficulty making quick decisions to drive or go for a walk alone may now be risky.

It might be difficult to restrict or take away our sense of independence when it comes to activities like driving and cooking. However, because safety is a major priority, it is critical to address these concerns as they emerge. While making these decisions, keep in mind that your loved one may no longer be able to detect what is best for them, but you can.

For example, taking the car away may elicit powerful emotions, but you must remain the voice of reason. The greatest thing you can do is start the conversation in a non-confrontational tone and be sympathetic to their feelings and reactions. Remember to give your loved one grace.

Act proactively as opposed to reactively
Dementia is a degenerative disease, therefore you should examine your loved one's needs on an ongoing basis. Caregivers must detect when a one-time incident becomes a pattern and act quickly to implement a solution. When caring for someone who has dementia, it is vital to be proactive rather than reactive. However, determining when to take these preventive actions is difficult.

If you're trying to establish whether your loved one requires more care or what more care entails, a home safety examination can help you assess:

* *Your loved one is at risk*
* *Are there any safety concerns?*
* *If there are any gaps in care*
* *What has to be done next*

Managing your parent's or loved one's care also involves a number of legal, financial, and medical issues to address. Getting an early start on them can be really beneficial. It is always more difficult to deal with a situation if you wait to implement the remedy until something happens. Delaying decision-making may limit your loved one's options in the future, but it may also represent a safety risk. I propose that you start planning for these medical and financial considerations as soon as your loved one receives the diagnosis.

Making decisions for others is always stressful, but reviewing your alternatives and making decisions ahead of time can help reduce the amount of stress you face in the long run. This is significant because, as a caregiver, you are likely to encounter a lot of it.

Know when to ask for help
Caring for someone with dementia can make it easy to neglect your own physical and emotional health. But don't forget about self-care.

Specifically, letting people assist you and being explicit about what the hell looks like are two of the best things you can do as a caregiver. Perhaps it means asking a family member to occasionally drive your loved one to a doctor's appointment or depending on a supermarket delivery service. Make the most of your time away by doing whatever it takes to unwind and refresh.

One thing I've noticed that caregivers struggle with cognitively is deciding whether to involve more people in the caring process and especially when to delegate to specialists. Doing so may feel like you're giving up on your loved one, which can elicit a wide range of conflicting feelings. Nonetheless, taking care of a loved one by yourself can be quite challenging.

Many dementia caregiver resources are available to assist you in your caregiving journey.

And, as it becomes evident that it is time for a care transition, keep reminding yourself that you are not alone.

Do not feel guilty about entrusting your loved one's care to specialists when the time comes. Relying on specialists can allow you to spend more quality time with your loved one, doing things you enjoy together rather than merely helping with day-to-day responsibilities.

While it is natural to want to care for your loved one for as long as possible, the unfortunate reality of dementia is that doing so may become dangerous for both of you. If the person with dementia wanders away or becomes lost, develops mobility or falling issues, exhibits extreme agitation or violence, or experiences any other change that causes you to be concerned about their or your own safety, a specialized memory care community may be the solution.

Specialized memory care provides dementia-trained staff and an environment that is expressly designed to help persons with dementia thrive.

Luckily, your loved one will move more smoothly from home to a memory care facility or between levels of care in a Life Plan Community if you have been helping them create regular routines. Typically, community workers will create a personalized plan of care that respects the individual's established habits and preferences, allowing them to continue doing the activities they enjoy in a safe and secure environment that provides them with peace of mind.